**ERIC WILLIAMS**

# Crumblin Herbs : A guide to herbal medicines and cures

*"Dedicated to all seekers of holistic well-being,
who embrace the wisdom of nature's healing gifts
and journey towards wellness with gratitude and mindfulness."*

# Contents

# Foreword

Welcome to the world of herbal health remedies, where ancient wisdom meets modern wellness. In these pages, you'll discover a treasure trove of natural solutions for common ailments, empowering you to take charge of your health in a holistic and sustainable way.

Herbal medicine has been practiced for centuries, passed down through generations as a testament to the healing power of plants. Today, as we navigate a world filled with synthetic medications and complex healthcare systems, the resurgence of interest in herbal remedies is a testament to our innate connection to nature and our quest for gentle, effective healing modalities.

This book is a comprehensive guide to herbal health remedies, covering a wide range of topics from creating your herbal medicine kit to exploring herbal teas, from managing pain to promoting mental wellness. Each chapter is a journey into the vast realm of botanical medicine, offering insights, recipes, and practical tips to integrate herbal remedies seamlessly into your lifestyle.

As you embark on this herbal journey, remember that herbal

medicine is not just about treating symptoms; it's about nurturing a relationship with nature, honoring the wisdom of traditional healing practices, and embracing a holistic approach to well-being. Whether you're seeking relief from a specific ailment, enhancing your daily self-care rituals, or simply curious about the wonders of herbalism, this book is your companion on the path to natural health and vitality.

May the knowledge and wisdom shared within these pages inspire and empower you on your journey to wellness.

Warm regards,

Eric K. Williams

# Preface

Herbal medicine is not just a collection of remedies; it's a doorway to a profound understanding of our interconnectedness with the natural world. In this book, we delve into the rich tapestry of herbal health remedies, weaving together ancient wisdom, modern science, and practical guidance to empower you on your wellness journey.

The resurgence of interest in herbal remedies reflects a growing recognition of the limitations of conventional medicine and a deep yearning for holistic approaches to health. As we navigate the complexities of modern life, it's essential to rediscover the healing treasures that nature has generously bestowed upon us.

This book is a labor of love, crafted with the intention of bridging the gap between traditional herbal knowledge and contemporary health needs. Each chapter is designed to be a roadmap, guiding you through the vast terrain of herbal medicine and offering practical strategies for incorporating herbal remedies into your daily life.

We begin by laying the foundation with an introduction to herbal remedies, understanding the basics of herbal medicine, and creating your herbal medicine kit. From there, we explore specific herbal solutions for common ailments, respiratory health, digestive disorders, skin conditions, mental wellness, women's health, men's health, children's health, pain management, stress, and anxiety.

Throughout these pages, you'll encounter a diverse array of herbs, each with its unique healing properties and therapeutic benefits. From the soothing aroma of lavender to the immune-boosting prowess of echinacea, every herb has a story to tell and a gift to offer.

As you embark on this journey, I encourage you to approach herbal medicine with an open heart and a curious mind. Embrace the wisdom of the plants, listen to your body's innate wisdom, and honor the interconnectedness of all living beings.

May this book serve as a trusted companion, guiding you towards greater well-being, vitality, and harmony with nature.

With gratitude and blessings,

Eric K. Williams

# Acknowledgement

Writing a book on herbal health remedies is a collaborative effort that draws upon the expertise, guidance, and support of numerous individuals and resources. I extend my heartfelt gratitude to everyone who contributed to the creation of this book and enriched its content with their knowledge, insights, and encouragement.

First and foremost, I would like to express my deepest appreciation to the herbalists, healers, and practitioners who have dedicated their lives to the study and practice of herbal medicine. Your wisdom, experience, and passion for plant-based healing have inspired the pages of this book and illuminated the path to natural wellness.

I am grateful to the researchers, authors, and educators whose work has contributed to the understanding of herbal medicine and its applications in modern health care. Your contributions to the field have paved the way for a greater appreciation of herbal remedies and their efficacy.

I extend my thanks to the botanical experts and suppliers who provide high-quality herbs, essential oils, and herbal products. Your commitment to sustainability, purity, and ethical sourcing ensures that readers have access to the finest ingredients for their herbal remedies.

I would like to acknowledge the editors, designers, and publishing professionals who contributed their expertise to bring this book to life. Your dedication to excellence and attention to detail have helped shape this work into its final form.

I am grateful to my family and friends for their unwavering support, encouragement, and understanding throughout the writing process. Your belief in this project and your encouragement kept me motivated and inspired to share the knowledge of herbal health remedies with others.

Lastly, I express my heartfelt appreciation to the readers who embark on this herbal journey. May the information and insights shared in this book empower you to embrace the healing power of nature and nurture a deeper connection to holistic well-being.

With gratitude,
Eric K. Williams

**One**

# Introduction to Herbal Remedies

Welcome to the fascinating world of herbal remedies, where ancient wisdom meets modern wellness. In this chapter, we'll embark on a journey to understand the roots of herbal medicine, explore its relevance in today's health landscape, and uncover the incredible potential of plant-based healing.

**Ancient Origins of Herbal Medicine**

Herbal medicine traces its roots back thousands of years to ancient civilizations such as the Egyptians, Greeks, Chinese, and Indigenous cultures around the world. These early healers relied on nature's bounty—plants, roots, bark, and flowers—to address a wide range of ailments. Their knowledge was passed down through generations, forming the basis of traditional herbal medicine systems that are still practiced today.

In ancient Egypt, healers used herbs like aloe vera for skin ailments and garlic for its antimicrobial properties. The Greeks, influenced by figures like Hippocrates, embraced herbalism as a fundamental part of their medical practices, recognizing the healing powers of plants like chamomile and peppermint.

Traditional Chinese Medicine (TCM) developed a sophisticated understanding of herbal remedies, categorizing herbs based on their energetic properties and using them in intricate formulas to restore balance and harmony in the body. Ginseng, astragalus, and reishi mushroom are just a few examples of revered Chinese herbs known for their adaptogenic and immune-boosting properties.

Indigenous cultures across the globe cultivated deep relationships with local plants, harnessing their healing properties for everything from wound care to spiritual ceremonies. Native American herbalism, for instance, utilized plants like echinacea and sage for their medicinal and ceremonial significance.

**Herbal Medicine in Modern Times**

Fast forward to the present day, and herbal medicine continues to thrive alongside conventional healthcare practices. In fact, there's been a resurgence of interest in herbal remedies as people seek natural alternatives to synthetic drugs and embrace holistic approaches to health and wellness.

One of the key attractions of herbal medicine is its emphasis on treating the root cause of illness rather than just addressing symptoms. Herbs work synergistically with the body's own healing mechanisms, supporting overall well-being and promoting long-term vitality.

Moreover, herbal remedies often have fewer side effects compared to pharmaceutical medications, making them appealing options for individuals looking to minimize adverse reactions while still achieving therapeutic benefits.

**The Science Behind Herbal Medicine**

While herbal medicine is deeply rooted in tradition and

# Two

# Understanding the Basics of Herbal Medicine

Welcome to the foundational chapter on herbal medicine, where we'll delve into the core principles, terminology, and practices that form the backbone of this ancient healing art. By understanding the basics of herbal medicine, you'll gain insight into how plants interact with the human body, how to identify and use medicinal herbs safely, and how to navigate the rich tapestry of herbal remedies available.

**The Language of Herbal Medicine**

Before we dive into the specifics, let's familiarize ourselves with some key terms and concepts used in herbalism:

1. **Active Compounds:** These are the bioactive molecules within plants that exert therapeutic effects on the body. Examples include curcumin in turmeric, menthol in peppermint, and hypericin in St. John's Wort.

2. **Actions and Properties:** Herbs are often classified based on their actions (what they do in the body) and properties (their inherent characteristics). For instance, an herb may have analgesic (pain-relieving) properties and be classified as a nervine (calming to the nervous system).

3. **Dosage Forms:** Herbal remedies come in various forms such as teas, tinctures, capsules, poultices, and salves. Each form has its advantages and considerations in terms of absorption, potency, and ease of use.

4. **Synergy:** Many herbalists believe in the concept of synergy, where the combined action of multiple herbs in a formula enhances their overall effectiveness. This is why herbal blends often yield better results than single herbs alone.

## How Herbs Interact with the Body

Herbs contain a diverse array of chemical compounds that interact with our bodies in complex ways. These interactions can include:

1. **Pharmacological Actions:** Herbs may mimic or modulate the effects of pharmaceutical drugs. For example, valerian root has sedative properties similar to certain prescription sleep aids.

2. **Nutritional Support:** Many herbs are rich in vitamins, minerals, and antioxidants that support overall health. Nettle leaf, for instance, is a nutrient-dense herb high in iron, calcium, and vitamin C.

3. **Modulating Body Systems:** Herbs can influence various body systems such as the immune system, digestive system, nervous system, and cardiovascular system. For

example, ginger is known for its digestive and anti-nausea properties.

4. **Adaptogenic Effects:** Adaptogens are a class of herbs that help the body adapt to stress and promote resilience. Examples include ashwagandha, rhodiola, and holy basil.

Understanding how herbs interact with the body is essential for using them effectively and safely.

**Identifying and Sourcing Medicinal Herbs**

One of the fundamental skills in herbal medicine is knowing how to identify and source high-quality herbs. Here are some guidelines:

1. **Botanical Identification:** Learn to identify herbs based on their botanical features such as leaves, flowers, stems, and roots. Field guides, herbal manuals, and online resources can be valuable tools.

2. **Quality and Purity:** Source herbs from reputable suppliers that prioritize quality, sustainability, and ethical harvesting practices. Look for organic certification and third-party testing for purity and potency.

3. **Growing Your Own:** Consider growing medicinal herbs in your garden or indoor pots. This not only ensures freshness but also deepens your connection to the plants and their healing properties.

4. **Wildcrafting:** If foraging for wild herbs, do so responsibly and ethically. Respect conservation guidelines, avoid endangered species, and only harvest from clean, uncontaminated areas.

**Preparing Herbal Remedies**

Once you have your medicinal herbs, you can prepare them in various forms to create herbal remedies. Here are some common methods:

1. **Herbal Teas:** Infuse dried or fresh herbs in hot water to make herbal teas. This simple method extracts the medicinal compounds and flavors of the herbs.
2. **Tinctures:** Tinctures are concentrated liquid extracts of herbs made by soaking them in alcohol or glycerin. They are potent and have a longer shelf life than teas.
3. **Decoctions:** Some herbs, particularly roots and barks, require simmering in water to extract their medicinal properties fully. This method is called decoction and is often used for tougher plant parts.
4. **Poultices and Compresses:** For topical applications, herbs can be used in poultices (herb paste applied to the skin) or compresses (herb-infused cloth applied to the skin).
5. **Herbal Oils and Salves:** Infuse herbs in carrier oils like olive oil or coconut oil to create herbal oils for massage or topical use. Herbal oils can also be solidified with beeswax to make healing salves.

## Safety Considerations

While herbal medicine is generally safe when used appropriately, it's essential to be aware of potential risks and contraindications. Here are some safety considerations:

1. **Allergies and Sensitivities:** Some individuals may be allergic or sensitive to certain herbs. Always start with small doses and observe any adverse reactions.

2. **Drug Interactions:** Certain herbs can interact with medications, either enhancing or reducing their effects. Consult a healthcare professional if you're taking medications alongside herbal remedies.

3. **Pregnancy and Lactation:** Some herbs are contraindicated during pregnancy and breastfeeding. Seek guidance from a qualified herbalist or healthcare provider for safe herbal use during these times.

4. **Quality and Contamination:** Ensure herbs are sourced from reputable suppliers to avoid contamination with pesticides, heavy metals, or other toxins.

By understanding the basics of herbal medicine—from how herbs interact with the body to proper identification, sourcing, and preparation—you'll be equipped to embark on a rewarding journey of holistic healing and wellness. In the chapters ahead, we'll delve deeper into specific herbs, ailments, and therapeutic protocols, empowering you to harness the power of nature's pharmacy for optimal health and vitality.

**Three**

# Creating Your Herbal Medicine Kit

Congratulations on taking the first steps toward building your herbal medicine kit! In this chapter, we'll guide you through the process of assembling a well-rounded collection of medicinal herbs, tools, and resources to support your journey into herbal healing. Whether you're a novice or seasoned herbal enthusiast, having a well-stocked herbal medicine kit ensures you're prepared to address a wide range of health concerns naturally and effectively.

**Essential Components of Your Herbal Medicine Kit**

1. **Medicinal Herbs:** Start by selecting a variety of medicinal herbs that address common health issues and align with your specific wellness goals. Consider herbs with diverse actions and properties, such as anti-inflammatory, immune-boosting, and calming herbs. Some versatile herbs to include are:

- **Echinacea:** Boosts the immune system and helps fight off colds and infections.
- **Calendula:** Soothes skin irritations, promotes wound healing, and has anti-inflammatory properties.
- **Chamomile:** Calms the nervous system, aids digestion, and promotes relaxation.
- **Peppermint:** Relieves digestive discomfort, eases headaches, and has a refreshing flavor for teas.
- **Lavender:** Supports relaxation, relieves stress and anxiety, and has antimicrobial properties.
- **Ginger:** Settles the stomach, reduces inflammation, and supports circulation.

1. **Storage Containers:** Choose containers that keep your herbs fresh and protected from light, moisture, and air. Options include glass jars, amber tincture bottles, and resealable bags. Label each container with the herb's name, date of purchase, and any relevant information (e.g., dosage, contraindications).
2. **Tools and Equipment:**

- **Mortar and Pestle:** For grinding herbs into powders or making herbal pastes.
- **Measuring Spoons and Cups:** Accurate measurements are essential for preparing herbal remedies.
- **Infusion Strainer or Tea Ball:** For brewing herbal teas and infusions.
- **Funnel:** Helps transfer powdered herbs or liquids into bottles without spillage.
- **Double Boiler or Crockpot:** For gently heating herbs in oils or making herbal infusions.

1. **Books and References:** Invest in reputable herbal books, guides, and online resources to expand your knowledge of medicinal herbs, herbal actions, and remedy formulations. Reliable sources provide valuable information on dosage, safety precautions, and herbal interactions.
2. **Labeling Supplies:** Keep a supply of labels, markers, and adhesive tags handy for labeling your herbal containers with clear and informative details. Include the herb's common and botanical name, parts used, preparation instructions, and any cautions or contraindications.

**Selecting and Sourcing Quality Herbs**

When choosing herbs for your medicine kit, prioritize quality, freshness, and sustainability. Here are some tips for selecting and sourcing herbs:

1. **Organic Certification:** Opt for organically grown or wildcrafted herbs whenever possible to avoid exposure to pesticides, herbicides, and other contaminants.
2. **Reputable Suppliers:** Purchase herbs from trusted suppliers with a reputation for quality, ethical sourcing practices, and transparency about their products' origins.
3. **Freshness and Potency:** Check the freshness and potency of herbs by examining their color, aroma, and texture. Store herbs in a cool, dark place to maintain their medicinal properties.
4. **Ethical Harvesting:** If wildcrafting herbs, follow ethical guidelines to ensure sustainability and respect for natural ecosystems. Harvest responsibly and only collect herbs from abundant, non-endangered species.

**Building a Herbal First Aid Kit**

In addition to your general herbal medicine kit, consider creating a herbal first aid kit for addressing common injuries, cuts, bruises, and minor ailments. Include the following items:

1. **Arnica Salve:** Soothes muscle aches, bruises, and sprains.
2. **Plantain Leaf Poultice:** Relieves insect bites, stings, and minor skin irritations.
3. **Activated Charcoal Powder:** Absorbs toxins in case of poisoning or digestive issues.
4. **Aloe Vera Gel:** Calms sunburns, minor burns, and skin inflammations.
5. **Comfrey Leaf Infused Oil:** Promotes wound healing and soothes skin rashes.

**Herbal Medicine Kit Maintenance**

Regularly maintain and update your herbal medicine kit to ensure freshness, potency, and effectiveness. Here are some maintenance tips:

1. **Check Expiry Dates:** Periodically check the expiration dates of herbs and herbal products in your kit. Discard any expired or degraded items and replace them with fresh supplies.
2. **Rotate Herbs:** Use a first-in, first-out approach to rotate your herbal inventory. This ensures you're consistently using fresh herbs and prevents herbs from losing their potency over time.
3. **Storage Conditions:** Store your herbal medicine kit in a cool, dry place away from direct sunlight and humidity. Consider using airtight containers or vacuum-sealed bags

for long-term storage.

4. **Documentation:** Keep a journal or digital record of your herbal remedies, including recipes, dosages, and outcomes. This documentation helps track your herbal experiences and adjustments for future reference.

## Customizing Your Herbal Medicine Kit

Your herbal medicine kit is a personalized collection tailored to your health needs and preferences. As you gain experience and knowledge, don't hesitate to add new herbs, experiment with different preparations, and refine your herbal formulations. Your kit evolves with you on your herbal journey, offering endless possibilities for natural healing and wellness.

By creating and maintaining a well-equipped herbal medicine kit, you're empowered to take charge of your health, explore the diverse benefits of medicinal herbs, and cultivate a deeper connection to nature's healing wisdom. In the chapters ahead, we'll explore specific herbs, remedies, and applications, guiding you toward a holistic approach to well-being through herbal medicine.

# Four

# Herbal Remedies for Common Ailments

In this chapter, we'll delve into the world of herbal remedies for everyday health concerns. From headaches to indigestion, these natural solutions harness the power of medicinal herbs to alleviate symptoms, promote healing, and support overall well-being. Let's explore some common ailments and the herbal remedies that can provide relief.

## 1. Headaches and Migraines

Headaches are a prevalent discomfort experienced by many people. Whether it's tension headaches, migraines, or sinus headaches, herbal remedies can offer soothing relief. Here are some herbs commonly used for headaches:

- **Feverfew (Tanacetum parthenium):** This herb is renowned for its ability to reduce the frequency and intensity of migraines. It works by inhibiting the release of

inflammatory substances in the brain.
- **Peppermint (Mentha piperita):** Peppermint contains menthol, which has a cooling effect and can help relax tense muscles in the head and neck, easing headache symptoms.
- **Willow Bark (Salix spp.):** Willow bark contains salicin, a compound similar to aspirin. It has analgesic and anti-inflammatory properties, making it effective for headache relief.

## 2. Digestive Discomfort

From indigestion to bloating, herbal remedies can support digestive health and ease discomfort after meals. Consider these herbs for digestive issues:

- **Ginger (Zingiber officinale):** Ginger is a digestive powerhouse, aiding in digestion, reducing nausea, and calming an upset stomach. It can be consumed as tea, added to meals, or taken in capsule form.
- **Peppermint (Mentha piperita):** Peppermint is not just for headaches; it's also excellent for relieving indigestion, gas, and bloating. Peppermint tea or oil can be particularly soothing.
- **Chamomile (Matricaria chamomilla):** Chamomile has anti-inflammatory and antispasmodic properties, making it beneficial for calming digestive spasms, reducing gas, and promoting overall digestive comfort.

## 3. Cold and Flu Symptoms

When cold and flu season arrives, herbal remedies can provide relief from congestion, sore throat, and other symptoms. These herbs are commonly used for colds and flu:

- **Echinacea (Echinacea purpurea):** Echinacea is a potent immune booster that can help shorten the duration and severity of colds and flu. It stimulates the immune system's response to viruses.
- **Elderberry (Sambucus nigra):** Elderberry is rich in antioxidants and has antiviral properties, making it effective against cold and flu viruses. Elderberry syrup is a popular remedy for respiratory symptoms.
- **Garlic (Allium sativum):** Garlic is a natural antimicrobial agent that can help fight off infections and support immune function. Raw garlic or garlic supplements are commonly used during cold and flu season.

## 4. Insomnia and Sleep Issues

Sleep is essential for overall health and well-being. Herbal remedies can promote relaxation, ease anxiety, and improve sleep quality. Here are some herbs for insomnia and sleep issues:

- **Valerian Root (Valeriana officinalis):** Valerian is a well-known herb for promoting relaxation and improving sleep quality. It's often used in herbal sleep aids and teas.
- **Chamomile (Matricaria chamomilla):** Chamomile's calming properties extend to promoting better sleep. A warm cup of chamomile tea before bedtime can help induce relaxation.
- **Lavender (Lavandula angustifolia):** Lavender is renowned for its soothing aroma, which can reduce anxiety and improve sleep. Use lavender essential oil in a diffuser or add a few drops to a warm bath.

## 5. Stress and Anxiety

In today's fast-paced world, stress and anxiety are common challenges. Herbal remedies offer natural ways to calm the mind and support emotional well-being. Consider these herbs for stress and anxiety:

- **Ashwagandha (Withania somnifera):** Ashwagandha is an adaptogenic herb that helps the body adapt to stress and promote balance. It can reduce cortisol levels and improve resilience to stressors.
- **Passionflower (Passiflora incarnata):** Passionflower has calming and sedative effects, making it useful for reducing anxiety, promoting relaxation, and improving sleep quality.
- **Lemon Balm (Melissa officinalis):** Lemon balm is a gentle nervine herb that soothes nervous tension, lifts mood, and promotes a sense of calm. It's often used in teas and tinctures for anxiety relief.

## 6. Minor Wounds and Skin Irritations

For cuts, scrapes, burns, and other minor wounds, herbal remedies can aid in healing, reduce inflammation, and prevent infection. Here are some herbs for minor wounds and skin irritations:

- **Calendula (Calendula officinalis):** Calendula is a potent wound healer with anti-inflammatory and antimicrobial properties. It's commonly used in salves, creams, and infused oils for skin injuries.
- **Comfrey (Symphytum officinale):** Comfrey is known for its rapid healing properties, particularly for bruises, sprains, and minor cuts. Use comfrey in poultices, salves,

or infused oils for topical application.

- **Plantain (Plantago major):** Plantain is a versatile herb that soothes insect bites, stings, rashes, and minor skin irritations. Its natural anti-inflammatory properties make it a valuable addition to your herbal first aid kit.

## 7. Allergies and Respiratory Issues

Seasonal allergies, asthma, and respiratory infections can be managed with herbal remedies that support respiratory health and ease allergy symptoms. Consider these herbs for allergies and respiratory issues:

- **Nettle Leaf (Urtica dioica):** Nettle leaf is a natural anti-histamine that reduces allergy symptoms such as sneezing, itching, and nasal congestion. It's available as a tea, tincture, or capsule.
- **Marshmallow Root (Althaea officinalis):** Marshmallow root has soothing and demulcent properties, making it effective for calming inflamed airways, reducing coughing, and easing sore throats.
- **Thyme (Thymus vulgaris):** Thyme is a powerful antimicrobial herb with expectorant properties, making it beneficial for respiratory infections, coughs, and congestion. Use thyme in teas or as a steam inhalation.

## Safety Considerations and Precautions

While herbal remedies are generally safe, it's essential to exercise caution and consult with a healthcare professional, especially if you have underlying health conditions, are pregnant or nursing, or are taking medications. Some herbs may interact with medications or have contraindications for certain populations.

When using herbal remedies:

- Start with small doses and observe any reactions.
- Research potential herb-drug interactions.
- Use herbs according to recommended dosages and guidelines.
- Discontinue use if you experience adverse effects and seek medical attention if needed.

## Conclusion

Herbal remedies offer effective and natural solutions for common ailments, providing relief while supporting overall health and well-being. By incorporating these herbs into your wellness routine, you can tap into the healing power of nature and experience the benefits of herbal medicine firsthand

# Five

# Herbal Remedies for Respiratory Health

Respiratory health is crucial for overall well-being, as it directly impacts our ability to breathe, oxygenate our bodies, and maintain vitality. In this chapter, we'll explore a range of herbal remedies specifically targeted at supporting respiratory health, addressing common issues such as congestion, coughs, allergies, asthma, and respiratory infections. These herbal allies can soothe inflamed airways, clear congestion, boost immunity, and promote optimal respiratory function.

**Understanding Respiratory Health**

Before delving into herbal remedies, let's briefly discuss the respiratory system and common respiratory ailments:

1. **Respiratory System Overview:** The respiratory system consists of organs such as the nose, throat, trachea, bronchi, and lungs, responsible for the intake of oxygen

and expulsion of carbon dioxide. It plays a vital role in oxygenation, immune defense, and maintaining acid-base balance in the body.

2. **Common Respiratory Ailments:**

- **Congestion:** Nasal congestion and sinus congestion can result from allergies, colds, or sinus infections, leading to difficulty breathing and discomfort.
- **Coughs:** Coughing is a reflex action that helps clear the airways of irritants, mucus, or pathogens. Persistent coughs can be due to respiratory infections, allergies, or asthma.
- **Asthma:** Asthma is a chronic respiratory condition characterized by inflammation and narrowing of the airways, leading to wheezing, shortness of breath, and coughing.
- **Respiratory Infections:** Viral and bacterial infections such as the common cold, flu, bronchitis, and pneumonia can affect the respiratory system, causing symptoms like coughing, congestion, and difficulty breathing.

Now, let's explore herbal remedies that can help alleviate these respiratory issues and promote lung health.

**1. Echinacea (Echinacea purpurea)**

Echinacea is a potent immune-boosting herb that supports respiratory health by enhancing the body's defense mechanisms against infections. It stimulates white blood cell activity, reduces inflammation, and shortens the duration of colds and respiratory infections. Echinacea is available in various forms, including teas, tinctures, capsules, and throat lozenges.

**2. Elderberry (Sambucus nigra)**

Elderberry is rich in antioxidants and has strong antiviral properties, making it an effective remedy for respiratory infections such as the flu and colds. Elderberry syrup or extract can reduce the severity and duration of symptoms by inhibiting viral replication and boosting immune function.

### 3. Thyme (Thymus vulgaris)

Thyme is a versatile herb with antimicrobial, expectorant, and bronchodilator properties, making it beneficial for respiratory health. Thyme tea or steam inhalation can help relieve congestion, coughs, and respiratory infections. It also supports the immune system and soothes inflamed airways.

### 4. Peppermint (Mentha piperita)

Peppermint is known for its cooling and decongestant properties, making it effective for relieving nasal congestion, sinus pressure, and respiratory discomfort. Peppermint tea, steam inhalation, or chest rubs with peppermint oil can help open up the airways, ease breathing, and soothe respiratory symptoms.

### 5. Licorice Root (Glycyrrhiza glabra)

Licorice root has expectorant and anti-inflammatory properties that make it useful for treating respiratory conditions such as bronchitis, coughs, and sore throats. It helps loosen mucus, reduce coughing, and soothe irritated throat tissues. Licorice root tea or decoctions can be consumed to support respiratory health.

### 6. Osha Root (Ligusticum porteri)

Osha root is a traditional Native American herb known for its respiratory benefits. It has antiviral, expectorant, and bronchodilator properties, making it effective for treating respiratory infections, asthma, and coughs. Osha root tinctures or teas can be used to alleviate respiratory symptoms and support lung function.

### 7. Mullein (Verbascum thapsus)

Mullein is a gentle yet effective herb for respiratory health, especially for soothing coughs, congestion, and respiratory irritation. Its mucilaginous properties help moisten and soothe dry, irritated airways, making it beneficial for conditions like bronchitis and asthma. Mullein leaf tea or herbal infusions are commonly used for respiratory support.

**8. Marshmallow Root (Althaea officinalis)**

Marshmallow root is another mucilaginous herb that provides soothing relief for respiratory issues. It forms a protective layer in the throat and respiratory tract, reducing irritation, coughing, and inflammation. Marshmallow root tea or lozenges can be used to alleviate sore throats and respiratory discomfort.

**Safety Considerations and Precautions**

While herbal remedies for respiratory health are generally safe, it's essential to consider individual sensitivities, allergies, and medical conditions. Here are some safety considerations and precautions:

1. **Allergies:** Some individuals may be allergic to certain herbs. Always start with small doses and monitor for any adverse reactions.

2. **Pregnancy and Nursing:** Consult a healthcare provider before using herbal remedies during pregnancy or while breastfeeding, as some herbs may have contraindications.

3. **Medication Interactions:** Certain herbs may interact with medications. If you're taking prescription medications, consult with a healthcare professional before using herbal remedies.

4. **Quality and Sourcing:** Choose high-quality, organic herbs from reputable suppliers to ensure purity, potency, and safety.

5. **Dosage:** Follow recommended dosages and guidelines for herbal remedies to avoid overuse or misuse.
6. **Professional Guidance:** If you have chronic respiratory conditions or severe symptoms, seek guidance from a qualified herbalist or healthcare provider for personalized advice and treatment options.

**Incorporating Herbal Remedies into Your Routine**

To incorporate herbal remedies for respiratory health into your daily routine:

1. **Herbal Teas:** Brew herbal teas using dried herbs or herbal tea blends specifically designed for respiratory support. Enjoy warm teas throughout the day to soothe throat irritation and ease congestion.
2. **Steam Inhalation:** Add a few drops of essential oils or dried herbs (such as thyme or eucalyptus) to hot water and inhale the steam to open up congested airways and relieve respiratory discomfort.
3. **Herbal Tinctures:** Take herbal tinctures formulated for respiratory health according to recommended dosages. Tinctures are concentrated extracts that can be easily added to water or juice.
4. **Herbal Syrups and Lozenges:** Use herbal syrups or lozenges containing respiratory-supportive herbs like licorice, elderberry, or marshmallow root to soothe sore throats and calm coughs.
5. **Herbal Chest Rubs:** Apply herbal chest rubs or balms containing respiratory herbs to the chest and throat area to provide localized relief from congestion and respiratory symptoms.

6. **Herbal Baths:** Add respiratory-supportive herbs like thyme, eucalyptus, or peppermint to your bathwater for inhalation benefits and overall respiratory comfort.

## Conclusion

Herbal remedies offer effective and natural support for respiratory health, addressing common ailments such as congestion, cough

# Six

# Herbal Solutions for Digestive Disorders

Digestive health plays a crucial role in overall well-being, as it impacts nutrient absorption, immune function, and even mood regulation. Digestive disorders such as indigestion, bloating, constipation, diarrhea, and irritable bowel syndrome (IBS) can significantly affect quality of life. In this chapter, we'll explore a range of herbal solutions specifically targeted at promoting digestive wellness, soothing digestive discomfort, and supporting optimal gut function.

**Understanding Digestive Disorders**

Before delving into herbal solutions, let's briefly discuss common digestive disorders and their symptoms:

1. **Indigestion:** Indigestion, also known as dyspepsia, is characterized by discomfort or pain in the upper abdomen, bloating, gas, and a feeling of fullness after meals. It can

be caused by overeating, spicy foods, stress, or underlying conditions.

2. **Bloating:** Bloating refers to a feeling of abdominal fullness, tightness, or swelling due to gas buildup in the digestive tract. It can be accompanied by discomfort, distension, and changes in bowel habits.

3. **Constipation:** Constipation is defined as infrequent bowel movements (less than three times per week), difficulty passing stools, straining during bowel movements, and hard or lumpy stools. It can be caused by inadequate fiber intake, dehydration, lack of physical activity, or certain medications.

4. **Diarrhea:** Diarrhea is characterized by loose, watery stools, frequent bowel movements, urgency, and abdominal cramping. It can be caused by infections, food intolerances, medications, or underlying gastrointestinal conditions.

5. **Irritable Bowel Syndrome (IBS):** IBS is a chronic digestive disorder characterized by abdominal pain, bloating, gas, diarrhea, constipation, or alternating bouts of diarrhea and constipation. It is often triggered by stress, diet, hormonal changes, or gut dysbiosis.

Now, let's explore herbal solutions that can help alleviate symptoms of these digestive disorders and promote digestive wellness.

### 1. Ginger (Zingiber officinale)

Ginger is a versatile herb with a long history of use in traditional medicine for digestive support. It has anti-inflammatory, carminative, and anti-nausea properties, making it beneficial for various digestive issues, including indigestion, bloating, nausea, and motion sickness. Ginger can be consumed as fresh ginger root, ginger tea, ginger capsules, or added to meals and beverages.

**2. Peppermint (Mentha piperita)**

Peppermint is well-known for its ability to soothe digestive discomfort and alleviate symptoms of indigestion, bloating, gas, and abdominal cramps. It has antispasmodic properties that relax the muscles of the digestive tract, easing cramping and promoting smoother digestion. Peppermint tea, peppermint oil capsules, or peppermint-infused foods can be used for digestive relief.

**3. Chamomile (Matricaria chamomilla)**

Chamomile is a gentle herb with calming, anti-inflammatory, and carminative properties, making it effective for soothing digestive upset, indigestion, gas, and bloating. Chamomile tea is a popular remedy for promoting relaxation, reducing stress-related digestive issues, and supporting overall digestive health.

**4. Licorice Root (Glycyrrhiza glabra)**

Licorice root is renowned for its demulcent, anti-inflammatory, and soothing properties, making it beneficial for treating various digestive disorders such as indigestion, heartburn, gastritis, and ulcers. It helps coat and protect the digestive tract, reducing inflammation, and promoting healing. Licorice root tea or deglycyrrhizinated licorice (DGL) supplements are commonly used for digestive support.

**5. Fennel (Foeniculum vulgare)**

Fennel seeds are rich in volatile oils that have carminative, anti-inflammatory, and digestive-stimulating effects, making them useful for relieving bloating, gas, and indigestion. Fennel tea, fennel seed capsules, or chewing fennel seeds after meals can aid in digestion, reduce bloating, and soothe digestive discomfort.

## 6. Marshmallow Root (Althaea officinalis)

Marshmallow root is a mucilaginous herb that forms a soothing gel-like substance when mixed with water. It has demulcent, anti-inflammatory, and protective effects on the digestive tract, making it beneficial for treating conditions such as gastritis, heartburn, indigestion, and ulcers. Marshmallow root tea, capsules, or powdered extracts can be used for digestive support.

## 7. Dandelion Root (Taraxacum officinale)

Dandelion root is a bitter herb that stimulates digestive secretions, enhances liver function, and supports overall digestion. It can improve bile flow, promote detoxification, and alleviate symptoms of indigestion, bloating, and sluggish digestion. Dandelion root tea, tinctures, or capsules are commonly used for digestive health.

## 8. Slippery Elm (Ulmus rubra)

Slippery elm is another mucilaginous herb that soothes and protects the digestive tract, making it beneficial for conditions like gastritis, heartburn, indigestion, and inflammatory bowel disorders. It forms a protective coating in the stomach and intestines, reducing inflammation and promoting healing. Slippery elm powder, capsules, or lozenges can be used for digestive support.

## 9. Turmeric (Curcuma longa)

Turmeric contains curcumin, a potent anti-inflammatory and antioxidant compound with digestive benefits. It helps reduce inflammation in the digestive tract, support liver function, and improve digestion. Turmeric can be consumed as fresh turmeric root, turmeric powder, turmeric capsules, or added to curries and beverages.

## 10. Artichoke Leaf (Cynara scolymus)

Artichoke leaf is rich in compounds that support liver function, bile production, and digestive health. It aids in digestion, reduces bloating, and supports gallbladder function, making it beneficial for indigestion, gas, and sluggish digestion. Artichoke leaf extract or teas can be used for digestive support.

### Safety Considerations and Precautions

While herbal remedies for digestive disorders are generally safe, it's essential to consider individual sensitivities, allergies, and medical conditions. Here are some safety considerations and precautions:

1. **Allergies:** Some individuals may be allergic to certain herbs. Always start with small doses and monitor for any adverse reactions.
2. **Pregnancy and Nursing:** Consult a healthcare provider before using herbal remedies during pregnancy or while breastfeeding, as some herbs may have contraindications.
3. **Medication Interactions:** Certain herbs may interact with medications. If you're taking prescription medications, consult with a healthcare professional before using herbal remedies.
4. **Chronic Conditions:** If you have chronic digestive conditions or severe symptoms, seek guidance from a qualified herbalist or healthcare provider for personalized advice and treatment options.
5. **Quality and Sourcing:** Choose high-quality, organic herbs from reputable suppliers to ensure purity, potency, and safety.
6. **Dosage:** Follow recommended dosages and guidelines for herbal remedies to avoid overuse or misuse.

**Incorporating Herbal Remedies into Your Routine**

To incorporate herbal solutions for digestive disorders into your daily routine:

1. **Herbal Teas:** Brew herbal teas using dried herbs or herbal tea blends specifically designed for digestive support. Enjoy warm teas after meals or between meals to aid digestion and soothe digestive discomfort.
2. **Herbal Tinctures:** Take herbal tinctures formulated for digestive health according to recommended dosages. Tinctures are concentrated extracts that can be easily added to water or juice.
3. **Herbal Capsules:** Use herbal capsules or tablets containing digestive-supportive herbs for convenient dosing and targeted digestive relief.
4. **Herbal Poultices:** Apply poultices or compresses containing herbal extracts or powdered herbs to the abdomen for localized relief from bloating, gas, or cramping.
5. **Herbal Cooking:** Incorporate digestive-friendly herbs and spices such as ginger, turmeric, fennel, and peppermint into your cooking and meal preparations to enhance digestion and flavor.
6. **Herbal Infusions:** Infuse digestive herbs in oil, vinegar, or honey to create flavorful and digestive-supportive condiments for salads, dressings, or marinades.

**Conclusion**

Herbal solutions offer effective and natural support for digestive disorders, promoting digestive wellness, soothing discomfort, and optimizing gut function. By incorporating these herbal remedies into your daily routine and adopting healthy lifestyle practices, you can experience improved digestion, reduced symptoms, and enhanced overall well-being. However, it's crucial to approach herbal remedies with knowledge, caution, and personalized guidance to ensure safe and effective use for your individual needs.

# Seven

# Herbal Remedies for Skin Conditions

Our skin serves as a protective barrier between our internal organs and the external environment. Skin conditions can range from mild irritations to chronic disorders, impacting both physical comfort and self-confidence. In this chapter, we'll explore herbal remedies that have been traditionally used to address various skin conditions, promoting healing, soothing discomfort, and restoring skin health.

**Understanding Common Skin Conditions**

Before diving into herbal remedies, let's understand some prevalent skin conditions and their characteristics:

1. **Acne:** Acne is a skin condition characterized by the presence of pimples, blackheads, whiteheads, and cysts. It often occurs due to clogged pores, excess oil production, hormonal fluctuations, and inflammation.

2. **Eczema (Dermatitis):** Eczema refers to a group of skin

conditions that cause redness, itching, inflammation, and sometimes blistering. It can be triggered by allergens, irritants, genetics, immune system dysfunction, or environmental factors.

3. **Psoriasis:** Psoriasis is an autoimmune condition that leads to the rapid growth of skin cells, resulting in red, scaly patches known as plaques. It can cause itching, discomfort, and changes in skin appearance.

4. **Dry Skin (Xerosis):** Dry skin is characterized by roughness, flakiness, tightness, and a lack of moisture. It can occur due to environmental factors, aging, dehydration, harsh soaps, or certain medical conditions.

5. **Minor Wounds and Irritations:** Minor wounds, cuts, scrapes, insect bites, rashes, and irritations are common skin issues that can result from accidents, environmental exposure, or allergic reactions.

## Herbal Remedies for Skin Conditions

1. **Aloe Vera (Aloe barbadensis):** Aloe vera is a versatile herb with cooling, anti-inflammatory, and wound-healing properties. It's commonly used to soothe sunburns, minor burns, cuts, insect bites, and skin irritations. Aloe vera gel can be applied directly to the affected area for relief and skin repair.

2. **Calendula (Calendula officinalis):** Calendula is renowned for its anti-inflammatory, antimicrobial, and skin-soothing effects. It's beneficial for eczema, dermatitis, minor wounds, rashes, and irritated skin. Calendula-infused oils, creams, or salves can be applied topically for healing and hydration.

3. **Chamomile (Matricaria chamomilla):** Chamomile has anti-inflammatory, antiseptic, and calming properties that make it useful for sensitive skin, eczema, dermatitis, and minor skin irritations. Chamomile tea bags can be steeped in warm water and applied as a compress or added to bathwater for skin relief.

4. **Lavender (Lavandula angustifolia):** Lavender is a soothing herb with anti-inflammatory, antimicrobial, and skin-regenerating effects. It helps calm irritated skin, reduce itching, and promote wound healing. Lavender essential oil can be diluted in a carrier oil and applied to the skin or added to bathwater for relaxation.

5. **Tea Tree (Melaleuca alternifolia):** Tea tree oil is a potent antimicrobial and anti-inflammatory herb that's beneficial for acne, fungal infections, insect bites, and minor wounds. It helps reduce bacteria, soothe inflammation, and promote clearer skin. Tea tree oil should be diluted before applying to the skin.

6. **Witch Hazel (Hamamelis virginiana):** Witch hazel is an astringent herb with anti-inflammatory and skin-toning properties. It can help reduce redness, soothe itching, and alleviate skin irritations such as eczema, psoriasis, and minor rashes. Witch hazel extract can be applied topically using a cotton pad or added to skincare products.

7. **Comfrey (Symphytum officinale):** Comfrey is known for its wound-healing, anti-inflammatory, and skin-repairing properties. It's beneficial for cuts, bruises, scrapes, minor burns, and skin irritations. Comfrey ointments, poultices, or infused oils can be applied to the skin for accelerated healing.

8. **Neem (Azadirachta indica):** Neem is a potent herb with

antibacterial, antifungal, and anti-inflammatory properties. It's effective against acne, eczema, psoriasis, and
fungal infections. Neem oil or neem-based creams can be
applied to affected areas for skin relief and protection.

9. **Turmeric (Curcuma longa):** Turmeric contains curcumin, a compound with anti-inflammatory, antioxidant,
and skin-healing properties. It's beneficial for acne,
eczema, psoriasis, and minor wounds. Turmeric paste
or turmeric-infused oils can be applied topically for skin
health and regeneration.

10. **Plantain (Plantago major):** Plantain is a soothing
herb with anti-inflammatory, antimicrobial, and wound-
healing effects. It's useful for insect bites, rashes, minor
wounds, and skin irritations. Plantain leaf poultices,
creams, or infused oils can be applied directly to the skin
for relief.

## Herbal Skin Care Tips

- **Patch Test:** Before using any herbal remedy on a large
  area of skin, perform a patch test to check for allergies or
  sensitivities.
- **Dilution:** Dilute potent essential oils like tea tree oil, neem
  oil, or lavender oil with a carrier oil to avoid skin irritation.
- **Sun Protection:** Use sunscreen or protective clothing
  when using photosensitive herbs like citrus oils.
- **Consistency:** Incorporate herbal remedies into your
  skincare routine consistently for best results.
- **Consultation:** If you have chronic skin conditions or
  severe symptoms, consult a dermatologist or herbalist for
  personalized advice.

## Conclusion

Herbal remedies offer gentle and effective solutions for a wide range of skin conditions, from acne and eczema to minor wounds and irritations. By harnessing the healing properties of medicinal herbs, you can promote skin health, alleviate discomfort, and restore your skin's natural balance. Experiment with different herbal remedies to find what works best for your skin type and concerns, and remember to practice patience and consistency for optimal results.

# Eight

# Harnessing Herbs for Mental Wellness

Mental wellness is an integral part of overall health, encompassing emotional, psychological, and cognitive well-being. Herbal remedies have been used for centuries to support mental wellness, alleviate stress, enhance mood, and promote relaxation. In this chapter, we'll explore a variety of herbs known for their calming, uplifting, and mood-balancing properties, offering natural support for mental health.

**Understanding Mental Wellness**

Before delving into herbal remedies, let's understand what mental wellness entails:

1. **Emotional Balance:** Mental wellness involves the ability to manage emotions effectively, cope with stress, and maintain a positive outlook on life.
2. **Cognitive Function:** It includes cognitive abilities such

as memory, concentration, problem-solving, and decision-making.

3. **Stress Management:** Mental wellness involves strategies and practices that help individuals cope with stressors, challenges, and life transitions.
4. **Mood Regulation:** It encompasses maintaining a stable and balanced mood, preventing mood swings, and managing symptoms of anxiety and depression.

## Herbs for Mental Wellness

1. **Ashwagandha (Withania somnifera):** Ashwagandha is an adaptogenic herb known for its stress-relieving and mood-balancing properties. It helps the body adapt to stress, reduces anxiety, and promotes relaxation. Ashwagandha supplements or teas can support mental well-being and overall resilience.
2. **Rhodiola (Rhodiola rosea):** Rhodiola is another adaptogenic herb that enhances mood, reduces fatigue, and improves cognitive function. It supports stress resilience, boosts energy levels, and promotes a sense of well-being. Rhodiola supplements or tinctures can be beneficial for mental clarity and focus.
3. **St. John's Wort (Hypericum perforatum):** St. John's Wort is well-known for its antidepressant and mood-stabilizing effects. It increases serotonin levels in the brain, alleviates symptoms of mild to moderate depression, and promotes emotional balance. St. John's Wort capsules or extracts should be used under professional guidance.
4. **Lemon Balm (Melissa officinalis):** Lemon balm is a calming herb that reduces anxiety, improves mood, and

promotes relaxation. It has mild sedative properties, making it beneficial for stress reduction and sleep support. Lemon balm tea or tinctures can be used to soothe nerves and enhance mental well-being.

5. **Chamomile (Matricaria chamomilla):** Chamomile is known for its calming and anti-anxiety effects. It reduces stress, promotes relaxation, and improves sleep quality. Chamomile tea is a popular choice for easing tension, calming nerves, and supporting mental wellness.

6. **Lavender (Lavandula angustifolia):** Lavender is a soothing herb that relieves anxiety, promotes relaxation, and improves sleep. Its aromatic properties have a calming effect on the mind and nervous system. Lavender essential oil can be used in aromatherapy, baths, or massage oils for mental well-being.

7. **Ginkgo Biloba (Ginkgo biloba):** Ginkgo biloba is known for its cognitive-enhancing properties. It improves memory, concentration, and cognitive function by enhancing blood flow to the brain and supporting brain health. Ginkgo biloba supplements are used to support mental clarity and focus.

8. **Holy Basil (Ocimum sanctum):** Holy basil, also known as tulsi, is an adaptogenic herb that reduces stress, boosts mood, and supports mental resilience. It has antioxidant and anti-inflammatory properties, making it beneficial for overall well-being. Holy basil tea or supplements can be used for stress management and mood support.

9. **Passionflower (Passiflora incarnata):** Passionflower is a calming herb that reduces anxiety, improves sleep quality, and promotes relaxation. It enhances the activity of gamma-aminobutyric acid (GABA), a neurotransmitter

that has calming effects on the brain. Passionflower tea or tinctures can be used for anxiety relief and stress management.

10. **Valerian Root (Valeriana officinalis):** Valerian root is a sedative herb that promotes relaxation, reduces anxiety, and improves sleep quality. It increases levels of GABA in the brain, leading to a calming effect. Valerian root supplements or teas can be used for anxiety relief and insomnia.

**Incorporating Herbal Remedies into Your Routine**

Here are some tips for incorporating herbal remedies into your routine for mental wellness:

1. **Herbal Teas:** Brew herbal teas using dried herbs or herbal tea blends designed for stress relief, mood enhancement, or relaxation. Enjoy a cup of herbal tea in the morning or evening to unwind and promote mental well-being.
2. **Herbal Supplements:** Take herbal supplements in capsule, tablet, or tincture form as directed by a healthcare professional or herbalist. Choose standardized herbal extracts for consistency and effectiveness.
3. **Aromatherapy:** Use essential oils in aromatherapy diffusers, inhalers, or massage oils to experience their calming, uplifting, or stress-relieving benefits. Essential oils like lavender, chamomile, and lemon balm are popular choices for aromatherapy.
4. **Herbal Baths:** Add dried herbs or herbal extracts to your bathwater for a relaxing and therapeutic experience. Epsom salts infused with lavender or chamomile essential oil can promote relaxation and ease muscle tension.

5. **Herbal Tinctures:** Take herbal tinctures formulated for mental wellness according to recommended dosages. Tinctures are concentrated extracts that can be easily absorbed and provide targeted benefits.
6. **Herbal Infusions:** Infuse herbs in oil, vinegar, or honey to create herbal-infused products for cooking, skincare, or wellness. For example, infuse lavender flowers in oil for a calming massage oil or culinary herb.
7. **Mindful Practices:** Combine herbal remedies with mindful practices such as meditation, deep breathing exercises, yoga, or journaling to enhance their effects on mental well-being.

## Safety Considerations and Precautions

- **Consultation:** Consult a healthcare professional or herbalist before using herbal remedies, especially if you have existing medical conditions, are pregnant or breastfeeding, or are taking medications.
- **Dosage:** Follow recommended dosages and guidelines for herbal supplements and extracts to avoid adverse effects or interactions.
- **Quality and Sourcing:** Choose high-quality, organic herbs and herbal products from reputable suppliers to ensure purity, potency, and safety.
- **Individual Sensitivities:** Be aware of individual sensitivities or allergies to certain herbs. Start with small doses and monitor for any adverse reactions.

## Conclusion

Herbal remedies offer valuable support for mental wellness,

helping to reduce stress, enhance mood, improve cognitive function, and promote relaxation. By incorporating these herbs into your daily routine through teas, supplements, aromatherapy, baths, and mindful practices, you can nurture your mental well-being naturally. Remember to prioritize self-care, seek professional guidance when needed, and listen to your body's signals for optimal mental health and balance.

# Nine

# Herbal Remedies for Women's Health

Women's health encompasses a wide range of physical, emotional, and reproductive concerns that evolve throughout different stages of life. Herbal remedies have long been utilized to support women's health, addressing issues such as hormonal balance, menstrual discomfort, menopause symptoms, reproductive wellness, and overall vitality. In this chapter, we'll explore a diverse array of herbs that have traditionally been used to promote women's health and well-being.

**Understanding Women's Health**

Women's health is a multifaceted aspect of overall wellness that includes:

1. **Hormonal Balance:** Maintaining balanced hormone levels is crucial for menstrual regularity, fertility, mood stability, and overall health.
2. **Menstrual Health:** Addressing menstrual discomfort, ir-

regular cycles, PMS symptoms, and hormonal fluctuations supports women's reproductive well-being.

3. **Reproductive Wellness:** Supporting reproductive organs, fertility, pregnancy, and postpartum recovery contributes to women's holistic health.

4. **Menopause Support:** Managing symptoms of menopause, such as hot flashes, mood swings, vaginal dryness, and hormonal changes, enhances quality of life during this transition.

5. **Emotional Well-Being:** Addressing emotional health, stress management, mood disorders, and mental wellness is vital for overall quality of life.

## Herbal Remedies for Women's Health

1. **Chasteberry (Vitex agnus-castus):** Chasteberry is an herb known for its ability to balance hormones, particularly in supporting menstrual regularity and alleviating symptoms of PMS (premenstrual syndrome). It can also be beneficial for managing symptoms of menopause.

2. **Red Raspberry Leaf (Rubus idaeus):** Red raspberry leaf is rich in nutrients and is commonly used to support women's reproductive health. It is believed to tone the uterus, improve fertility, ease menstrual cramps, and support a healthy pregnancy.

3. **Dong Quai (Angelica sinensis):** Dong quai is an herb widely used in Traditional Chinese Medicine to support women's health. It is believed to regulate menstrual cycles, alleviate menstrual pain, and support hormonal balance. Dong quai is often used in combination with other herbs for maximum benefits.

4. **Black Cohosh (Actaea racemosa):** Black cohosh is a popular herb for managing symptoms of menopause, such as hot flashes, night sweats, mood swings, and vaginal dryness. It has estrogen-like effects that can help balance hormonal changes during menopause.

5. **Evening Primrose Oil (Oenothera biennis):** Evening primrose oil is rich in gamma-linolenic acid (GLA), an omega-6 fatty acid that supports hormonal balance and may help alleviate symptoms of PMS and menopause, such as breast tenderness, mood swings, and bloating.

6. **Wild Yam (Dioscorea villosa):** Wild yam is often used as a natural alternative to hormone therapy. It contains diosgenin, a compound that can be converted into progesterone, supporting hormonal balance and easing symptoms related to menstruation and menopause.

7. **Nettle (Urtica dioica):** Nettle is a nutrient-rich herb that supports overall health, including women's reproductive health. It is high in iron, which can be beneficial for women with heavy menstrual bleeding or iron-deficiency anemia. Nettle tea or supplements provide nourishment and support.

8. **Ginger (Zingiber officinale):** Ginger is a warming herb that can help alleviate menstrual cramps, nausea, and digestive discomfort commonly associated with menstruation. It has anti-inflammatory properties that may reduce pain and inflammation.

9. **Motherwort (Leonurus cardiaca):** Motherwort is often used to support menstrual health, ease menstrual cramps, and regulate irregular periods. It is also beneficial for managing stress and anxiety, promoting emotional well-being.

10. **Saw Palmetto (Serenoa repens):** Saw palmetto is primarily known for its use in supporting prostate health in men, but it can also be beneficial for women. It may help regulate hormonal balance and support urinary tract health.

## Incorporating Herbal Remedies into Women's Health Routine

1. **Herbal Teas:** Brew herbal teas using single herbs or herbal blends specifically formulated for women's health. Enjoy herbal teas daily or during times of menstrual discomfort or hormonal fluctuations.
2. **Herbal Supplements:** Take herbal supplements in capsule, tablet, or tincture form as directed by a healthcare provider or herbalist. Choose reputable brands and follow recommended dosages.
3. **Herbal Baths:** Add herbal extracts, such as chamomile, lavender, or calendula, to your bathwater for relaxation, stress relief, and skin nourishment.
4. **Herbal Infusions:** Create herbal infusions by steeping herbs in oil, vinegar, or honey. Use infused oils for massage, skincare, or culinary purposes.
5. **Aromatherapy:** Use essential oils such as lavender, clary sage, or geranium in aromatherapy diffusers, baths, or massage oils to promote relaxation, balance hormones, and uplift mood.
6. **Herbal Poultices:** Apply herbal poultices or compresses containing herbs like chamomile, ginger, or comfrey to the abdomen or lower back to ease menstrual cramps and discomfort.

## Safety Considerations and Precautions

- **Consultation:** Consult with a healthcare professional or herbalist before using herbal remedies, especially if you are pregnant, breastfeeding, have underlying health conditions, or are taking medications.
- **Quality and Sourcing:** Choose high-quality, organic herbs and herbal products from reputable suppliers to ensure purity and potency.
- **Dosage:** Follow recommended dosages and guidelines for herbal supplements to avoid adverse effects or interactions.
- **Individual Sensitivities:** Be aware of individual sensitivities or allergies to certain herbs. Start with small doses and monitor for any adverse reactions.

## Conclusion

Herbal remedies offer valuable support for women's health throughout various stages of life, from menstrual wellness to menopause transition and overall reproductive well-being. By incorporating these herbs into daily routines through teas, supplements, baths, and mindful practices, women can nurture their health, balance hormones, ease discomfort, and promote emotional well-being naturally. Remember to prioritize self-care, seek professional guidance when needed, and listen to your body's signals for optimal women's health and vitality.

# Ten

# Herbal Support for Men's Health

Men's health encompasses a wide range of physical, emotional, and reproductive concerns that evolve throughout different stages of life. Herbal remedies have been used for centuries to support men's health, addressing issues such as hormonal balance, prostate health, sexual wellness, cardiovascular health, and overall vitality. In this chapter, we'll explore a diverse array of herbs that have traditionally been used to promote men's health and well-being.

**Understanding Men's Health**

Men's health includes various aspects such as:

1. **Hormonal Balance:** Maintaining optimal hormone levels, especially testosterone, is crucial for men's physical and emotional well-being.
2. **Prostate Health:** Supporting prostate function and addressing issues such as benign prostatic hyperplasia (BPH)

or prostate inflammation is essential for men's reproductive health.

3. **Sexual Wellness:** Enhancing libido, erectile function, and overall sexual performance contributes to men's quality of life and confidence.

4. **Cardiovascular Health:** Supporting heart health, blood pressure regulation, and cholesterol levels is vital for preventing cardiovascular diseases.

5. **Emotional Well-Being:** Addressing stress management, mental health, and emotional resilience is important for overall health and wellness.

## Herbal Remedies for Men's Health

1. **Saw Palmetto (Serenoa repens):** Saw palmetto is commonly used to support prostate health and reduce symptoms of benign prostatic hyperplasia (BPH), such as frequent urination, urinary urgency, and incomplete bladder emptying. It works by inhibiting the enzyme responsible for converting testosterone to dihydrotestosterone (DHT), which contributes to prostate enlargement.

2. **Tribulus Terrestris:** Tribulus terrestris is known for its potential to boost testosterone levels naturally. It may improve libido, enhance muscle strength and endurance, and support reproductive health in men.

3. **Horny Goat Weed (Epimedium):** Horny goat weed is a traditional Chinese herb used to improve erectile function, increase libido, and enhance sexual performance. It contains icariin, a compound that promotes blood flow to the genital area, supporting healthy erections.

4. **Ginseng (Panax ginseng):** Ginseng is an adaptogenic

herb that supports overall vitality, energy levels, and immune function. It may also improve erectile function, increase sperm count and motility, and enhance sexual performance.

5. **Maca Root (Lepidium meyenii):** Maca root is a Peruvian herb known for its aphrodisiac properties and ability to support hormonal balance. It may improve libido, increase sperm production, and reduce symptoms of erectile dysfunction.

6. **Ashwagandha (Withania somnifera):** Ashwagandha is an adaptogenic herb that helps reduce stress, improve energy levels, and support hormonal balance. It may enhance testosterone levels, boost libido, and improve overall sexual health in men.

7. **Nettle Root (Urtica dioica):** Nettle root is beneficial for prostate health and may help reduce symptoms of BPH. It works by inhibiting the conversion of testosterone to DHT and has anti-inflammatory properties that support urinary tract health.

8. **Pumpkin Seed (Cucurbita pepo):** Pumpkin seeds are rich in zinc, which is essential for prostate health, testosterone production, and sperm quality. Consuming pumpkin seeds or pumpkin seed oil may support overall reproductive wellness in men.

9. **Ginkgo Biloba (Ginkgo biloba):** Ginkgo biloba is known for its ability to improve blood circulation, including to the genital area. It may enhance erectile function, increase libido, and improve overall sexual performance.

10. **Yohimbe Bark (Pausinystalia yohimbe):** Yohimbe bark is used as a natural remedy for erectile dysfunction and sexual performance issues. It contains yohimbine, a

compound that dilates blood vessels and improves blood flow to the penis, supporting erections.

**Incorporating Herbal Remedies into Men's Health Routine**

1. **Herbal Supplements:** Take herbal supplements in capsule, tablet, or tincture form as directed by a healthcare provider or herbalist. Choose high-quality products from reputable brands.
2. **Herbal Teas:** Brew herbal teas using single herbs or herbal blends designed for men's health. Enjoy herbal teas daily for their therapeutic benefits.
3. **Dietary Changes:** Incorporate foods rich in nutrients that support men's health, such as zinc-rich foods (pumpkin seeds, oysters), antioxidant-rich fruits and vegetables, and healthy fats (omega-3 fatty acids from fish, flaxseeds).
4. **Physical Activity:** Engage in regular exercise and physical activity to support overall health, improve circulation, and boost energy levels.
5. **Stress Management:** Practice stress-reducing techniques such as meditation, deep breathing exercises, yoga, or hobbies that promote relaxation and emotional well-being.
6. **Regular Check-ups:** Schedule regular check-ups with a healthcare provider to monitor and address any underlying health concerns or conditions.

**Safety Considerations and Precautions**

- **Consultation:** Consult with a healthcare professional or herbalist before using herbal remedies, especially if you have underlying health conditions, are taking medications, or have specific concerns about prostate health or sexual function.

- **Dosage:** Follow recommended dosages and guidelines for herbal supplements to avoid adverse effects or interactions.
- **Quality and Sourcing:** Choose high-quality, organic herbs and herbal products from reputable suppliers to ensure purity and potency.
- **Individual Sensitivities:** Be aware of individual sensitivities or allergies to certain herbs. Start with small doses and monitor for any adverse reactions.

**Conclusion**

Herbal remedies offer valuable support for men's health, addressing issues such as prostate health, hormonal balance, sexual wellness, cardiovascular health, and overall vitality. By incorporating these herbs into daily routines through supplements, teas, dietary choices, physical activity, and stress management techniques, men can nurture their health, support reproductive wellness, and enhance overall well-being naturally. Remember to prioritize self-care, seek professional guidance when needed, and listen to your body's signals for optimal men's health and vitality.

# Eleven

# Natural Remedies for Children's Health

Children's health is a top priority for parents and caregivers, and natural remedies play a significant role in supporting their well-being. From common childhood ailments to promoting overall growth and development, natural remedies offer gentle and effective solutions. In this chapter, we'll explore a variety of natural remedies that are safe and beneficial for children's health, focusing on maintaining their physical, emotional, and immune system wellness.

**Understanding Children's Health**

Children's health encompasses a range of aspects, including:

1. **Physical Health:** Supporting growth, development, nutrition, and overall physical well-being.
2. **Emotional Well-Being:** Nurturing mental health, emotional resilience, and coping skills.

3. **Immune System Support:** Strengthening the immune system to prevent illness and promote faster recovery.
4. **Common Childhood Ailments:** Addressing common issues such as colds, fevers, coughs, allergies, and skin irritations.
5. **Holistic Wellness:** Promoting a balanced lifestyle that includes healthy nutrition, regular physical activity, adequate sleep, and emotional support.

## Natural Remedies for Children's Health

1. **Elderberry (Sambucus nigra):** Elderberry syrup is a popular natural remedy for boosting the immune system and fighting off colds and flu. It is rich in antioxidants and has antiviral properties that can help reduce the duration and severity of illnesses.
2. **Honey:** Honey is a soothing and natural cough remedy for children over one year old. It can be added to warm herbal teas or taken by the spoonful to ease coughs and throat irritation.
3. **Chamomile Tea:** Chamomile tea is calming and can help children relax, reduce anxiety, and improve sleep quality. It is safe for children and can be consumed before bedtime to promote a peaceful sleep.
4. **Probiotics:** Probiotics are beneficial bacteria that support digestive health and strengthen the immune system. They can be found in fermented foods like yogurt or taken as supplements for children.
5. **Echinacea:** Echinacea is an herb known for its immune-boosting properties. It can help prevent colds and shorten the duration of illnesses when taken at the onset of

symptoms.

6. **Ginger:** Ginger can be used to ease digestive discomfort, nausea, and motion sickness in children. It can be added to teas, soups, or smoothies in small amounts.

7. **Calendula Cream:** Calendula cream is soothing and can be applied topically to minor cuts, scrapes, insect bites, and rashes. It has anti-inflammatory and antimicrobial properties that promote skin healing.

8. **Lavender Essential Oil:** Lavender essential oil is calming and can be used in a diffuser to create a relaxing environment for children. It can also be diluted in a carrier oil and applied topically to promote sleep or soothe skin irritations.

9. **Arnica Gel:** Arnica gel is a natural remedy for bruises, muscle soreness, and minor injuries. It can be applied externally to affected areas to reduce pain and inflammation.

10. **Omega-3 Fatty Acids:** Omega-3 fatty acids, found in fish oil or flaxseed oil supplements, support brain development, cognitive function, and overall health in children.

**Incorporating Natural Remedies into Children's Health Routine**

1. **Healthy Diet:** Encourage a balanced diet rich in fruits, vegetables, whole grains, lean proteins, and healthy fats to support overall health and immune function.

2. **Regular Physical Activity:** Promote regular physical activity and outdoor play to strengthen muscles, bones, and cardiovascular health in children.

3. **Adequate Sleep:** Ensure children get enough sleep according to their age group, as adequate sleep is crucial for

growth, development, and immune system function.

4. **Emotional Support:** Create a nurturing and supportive environment that includes open communication, positive reinforcement, and stress-reducing activities for emotional well-being.
5. **Limit Sugar and Processed Foods:** Minimize consumption of sugary snacks, sodas, and processed foods, as they can weaken the immune system and contribute to health issues.
6. **Hydration:** Encourage children to drink plenty of water throughout the day to stay hydrated and support overall health.

## Safety Considerations and Precautions

- **Age Appropriateness:** Consider the age and developmental stage of the child when using natural remedies and consult with a healthcare provider for guidance.
- **Dosage:** Follow recommended dosages and guidelines for natural remedies to ensure safety and effectiveness.
- **Allergies:** Be aware of any allergies or sensitivities the child may have to certain herbs or ingredients.
- **Professional Advice:** Consult with a pediatrician or healthcare provider before using new natural remedies, especially if the child has underlying health conditions or is taking medications.

## Conclusion

Natural remedies offer valuable support for children's health, providing safe and effective solutions for common ailments, immune system support, emotional well-being, and overall wellness. By incorporating these remedies into children's daily routines alongside healthy lifestyle habits, parents and caregivers can nurture their well-being, promote resilience, and support optimal growth and development. Remember to prioritize safety, consult with healthcare professionals when needed, and empower children to take an active role in their health and wellness journey.

# Twelve

# Herbal Solutions for Pain Management

Pain is a complex and challenging experience that can affect various aspects of life, from physical well-being to emotional and mental health. While conventional pain management approaches often rely on medications, herbal solutions offer natural alternatives that can complement traditional treatments or be used independently. In this chapter, we'll explore a diverse range of herbs known for their pain-relieving properties and how they can be effectively utilized for managing different types of pain.

**Understanding Pain Management**

Pain can be classified into different categories based on its origin, duration, and intensity:

1. **Acute Pain:** Short-term pain usually caused by injury, surgery, or illness. It typically resolves as the underlying

cause heals.

2. **Chronic Pain:** Persistent pain lasting beyond the normal healing time, often lasting for weeks, months, or even years. Chronic pain can be challenging to manage and may require a multimodal approach.

3. **Neuropathic Pain:** Pain resulting from damage or dysfunction of the nervous system, leading to shooting, burning, or tingling sensations. Conditions like neuropathy, sciatica, or nerve compression can cause neuropathic pain.

4. **Inflammatory Pain:** Pain associated with inflammation, such as arthritis, joint pain, or muscle soreness. Inflammatory pain is often accompanied by swelling, redness, and stiffness.

## Herbal Solutions for Pain Management

1. **Turmeric (Curcuma longa):** Turmeric contains curcumin, a potent anti-inflammatory compound that can help reduce pain associated with inflammation, such as arthritis, joint pain, and muscle soreness. It also has antioxidant properties that support overall health.

2. **Ginger (Zingiber officinale):** Ginger is another herb with anti-inflammatory properties that can alleviate pain and reduce inflammation in conditions like osteoarthritis, rheumatoid arthritis, and muscle strains. It can be consumed as a tea, added to meals, or taken as a supplement.

3. **White Willow Bark (Salix alba):** White willow bark contains salicin, a compound similar to aspirin, which has analgesic and anti-inflammatory effects. It can be used to relieve headaches, muscle pain, and joint discomfort.

4. **Arnica (Arnica montana):** Arnica is commonly used

topically in the form of gels, creams, or ointments to reduce pain, swelling, and bruising associated with injuries, sprains, and muscle strains. It has anti-inflammatory and analgesic properties.

5. **Capsaicin (Capsicum annuum):** Capsaicin is derived from chili peppers and is often used in topical creams or patches to alleviate pain related to arthritis, neuropathy, and muscle soreness. It works by desensitizing pain receptors.

6. **Valerian Root (Valeriana officinalis):** Valerian root is known for its calming and sedative effects, making it useful for relieving tension headaches, muscle spasms, and general pain associated with stress or anxiety.

7. **Boswellia (Boswellia serrata):** Boswellia resin contains compounds that have anti-inflammatory properties and can help reduce pain and improve mobility in conditions like osteoarthritis and rheumatoid arthritis.

8. **St. John's Wort (Hypericum perforatum):** St. John's Wort is traditionally used for its mood-enhancing properties, but it also has mild analgesic effects that can help alleviate nerve pain, muscle tension, and headaches.

9. **Devil's Claw (Harpagophytum procumbens):** Devil's claw is used for its anti-inflammatory and pain-relieving properties, particularly in conditions like arthritis, back pain, and tendonitis. It can be taken as a supplement or used topically in creams.

10. **Kratom (Mitragyna speciosa):** Kratom leaves contain alkaloids that have pain-relieving and mood-enhancing effects. It is used traditionally to manage chronic pain, but its use should be approached cautiously due to potential side effects and dependency issues.

## Incorporating Herbal Solutions for Pain Management

1. **Consultation:** Consult with a healthcare provider or herbalist before starting any herbal remedies, especially if you have underlying health conditions, are pregnant or breastfeeding, or are taking medications.
2. **Dosage and Formulation:** Follow recommended dosages and guidelines for herbal supplements or preparations. Choose high-quality products from reputable sources.
3. **Topical Application:** For localized pain, consider using herbal creams, ointments, or oils directly on the affected area. Massage gently for better absorption and relief.
4. **Internal Use:** Some herbs can be consumed internally as teas, capsules, tinctures, or extracts. Follow the instructions on the product label or seek guidance from a healthcare professional.
5. **Combination Therapy:** Herbal remedies can be used in combination with conventional treatments, physical therapy, relaxation techniques, and lifestyle modifications for comprehensive pain management.

## Safety Considerations and Precautions

- **Individual Sensitivities:** Be aware of individual sensitivities or allergies to certain herbs. Start with small doses and monitor for any adverse reactions.
- **Quality and Sourcing:** Choose high-quality, organic herbs and herbal products from reputable suppliers to ensure purity, potency, and safety.
- **Professional Advice:** Seek professional advice before

using herbal remedies, especially for chronic or severe pain conditions. Herbal remedies should not replace medical treatment when necessary.

## Conclusion

Herbal solutions offer valuable options for pain management, providing natural alternatives to conventional medications for various types of pain. By understanding the properties and benefits of different herbs

# Thirteen

# Herbal Remedies for Stress and Anxiety

In today's fast-paced and demanding world, stress and anxiety have become prevalent issues affecting millions of people. While there are various approaches to managing stress and anxiety, herbal remedies offer a natural and holistic way to promote relaxation, calmness, and emotional well-being. In this chapter, we'll explore a range of herbs known for their stress-relieving and anxiety-reducing properties, providing valuable insights into incorporating herbal remedies into your lifestyle for greater mental wellness.

**Understanding Stress and Anxiety**

Stress is the body's response to challenging or threatening situations, triggering a cascade of physiological and psychological responses. While some level of stress is normal and even beneficial in certain situations, chronic stress can have detrimental effects on physical, emotional, and mental health.

Anxiety, on the other hand, is a persistent feeling of worry, fear, or unease that can range from mild to severe. It can be triggered by various factors such as work pressure, relationship issues, financial concerns, or traumatic experiences.

**Herbal Remedies for Stress and Anxiety**

1. **Lavender (Lavandula angustifolia):** Lavender is perhaps one of the most well-known herbs for promoting relaxation and reducing anxiety. Its calming aroma and soothing properties make it effective in alleviating stress, improving sleep quality, and enhancing overall well-being. You can use lavender essential oil in aromatherapy, add dried lavender flowers to teas, or use lavender-infused products for a calming effect.

2. **Chamomile (Matricaria chamomilla):** Chamomile is another herb renowned for its calming and sedative effects. It can help reduce anxiety, promote relaxation, and improve sleep quality. Chamomile tea is a popular choice for easing stress and nervousness, particularly before bedtime.

3. **Ashwagandha (Withania somnifera):** Ashwagandha is an adaptogenic herb that helps the body cope with stress more effectively. It can reduce cortisol levels (the stress hormone), improve resilience to stressors, and promote a sense of calmness. Ashwagandha supplements or powders are commonly used to support stress management.

4. **Passionflower (Passiflora incarnata):** Passionflower has mild sedative and anxiolytic (anxiety-reducing) properties, making it beneficial for alleviating symptoms of anxiety, restlessness, and insomnia. Passionflower tea or supplements can be used to promote relaxation and mental

well-being.

5. **Valerian Root (Valeriana officinalis):** Valerian root is a calming herb that can help reduce anxiety, improve sleep quality, and promote relaxation. It works by increasing levels of gamma-aminobutyric acid (GABA), a neurotransmitter that has calming effects on the brain. Valerian root supplements or teas can be used for stress relief and insomnia.

6. **Rhodiola (Rhodiola rosea):** Rhodiola is an adaptogenic herb that enhances resilience to stress, boosts mood, and improves cognitive function. It can reduce symptoms of stress and fatigue, increase energy levels, and support overall mental well-being. Rhodiola supplements are often used for stress management and mood enhancement.

7. **Holy Basil (Ocimum sanctum):** Holy basil, also known as tulsi, is an adaptogenic herb with stress-relieving properties. It helps reduce cortisol levels, improve energy levels, and promote emotional balance. Holy basil tea or supplements can be beneficial for managing stress and anxiety.

8. **Lemon Balm (Melissa officinalis):** Lemon balm is a calming herb that reduces anxiety, promotes relaxation, and improves mood. It has mild sedative properties, making it useful for stress reduction, sleep support, and overall mental wellness. Lemon balm tea or tinctures can be used for calming effects.

9. **Ginkgo Biloba (Ginkgo biloba):** Ginkgo biloba is known for its cognitive-enhancing properties, but it also has benefits for stress management. It improves blood flow to the brain, supports cognitive function, and may reduce symptoms of anxiety and stress. Ginkgo biloba supple-

ments are used to enhance mental clarity and resilience to stress.

10. **Kava Kava (Piper methysticum):** Kava kava is a traditional herb from the South Pacific known for its calming and anxiety-reducing effects. It interacts with GABA receptors in the brain, producing a relaxing and tranquilizing effect. Kava supplements or extracts should be used cautiously and under professional guidance due to potential side effects.

## Incorporating Herbal Remedies into Your Routine

1. **Herbal Teas:** Brew herbal teas using single herbs or blends designed for stress relief and anxiety reduction. Enjoy a cup of herbal tea daily or during stressful moments to promote relaxation.

2. **Herbal Supplements:** Take herbal supplements in capsule, tablet, or tincture form as directed by a healthcare professional or herbalist. Choose reputable brands and follow recommended dosages.

3. **Aromatherapy:** Use essential oils like lavender, chamomile, or lemon balm in aromatherapy diffusers, massage oils, or baths to create a calming atmosphere and reduce stress.

4. **Herbal Baths:** Add dried herbs such as lavender, chamomile, or rose petals to your bathwater for a relaxing and soothing experience. The aromatic properties of herbs can help calm the mind and body.

5. **Mindfulness Practices:** Combine herbal remedies with mindfulness techniques such as meditation, deep breathing exercises, yoga, or tai chi to enhance their stress-

relieving effects and promote overall well-being.

**Safety Considerations and Precautions**

- **Consultation:** Consult with a healthcare professional or herbalist before using herbal remedies, especially if you have underlying health conditions, are pregnant or breastfeeding, or are taking medications.
- **Dosage:** Follow recommended dosages and guidelines for herbal supplements and extracts to avoid adverse effects or interactions.
- **Quality and Sourcing:** Choose high-quality, organic herbs and herbal products from reputable suppliers to ensure purity, potency, and safety.
- **Individual Sensitivities:** Be aware of individual sensitivities or allergies to certain herbs. Start with small doses and monitor for any adverse reactions.

**Conclusion**

Herbal remedies offer valuable support for managing stress and anxiety, promoting relaxation, calmness, and emotional well-being naturally. By incorporating these herbs into daily routines through teas, supplements, aromatherapy, baths, and mindfulness practices, individuals can reduce stress levels, enhance resilience, and improve overall mental wellness. Remember to prioritize self-care, seek professional guidance when needed, and embrace holistic approaches to stress management for long-term well-being.

# Fourteen

# Exploring Herbal Teas and Infusions

Herbal teas and infusions have been cherished for centuries across various cultures for their soothing, healing, and refreshing properties. From promoting relaxation to supporting digestion and boosting immunity, herbal teas offer a diverse array of flavors and benefits. In this chapter, we'll delve into the world of herbal teas and infusions, exploring different herbs, their health benefits, brewing techniques, and tips for creating delightful herbal beverages.

**Understanding Herbal Teas and Infusions**

Herbal teas, also known as tisanes, are beverages made from steeping dried herbs, flowers, fruits, or spices in hot water. Unlike true teas (green, black, white, oolong) derived from the Camellia sinensis plant, herbal teas do not contain caffeine and are caffeine-free alternatives for those seeking a soothing beverage.

Infusions, on the other hand, refer to the process of extracting flavors, aromas, and beneficial compounds from herbs or botanicals by steeping them in hot water. Infusions can be made with various ingredients, including herbs, fruits, flowers, and spices, creating flavorful and aromatic beverages.

**Health Benefits of Herbal Teas and Infusions**

1. **Promoting Relaxation:** Many herbs such as chamomile, lavender, and lemon balm have calming properties that help reduce stress, anxiety, and promote relaxation.
2. **Digestive Support:** Herbs like peppermint, ginger, fennel, and dandelion root can aid digestion, soothe stomach discomfort, alleviate bloating, and support overall digestive health.
3. **Immune Boost:** Certain herbs such as echinacea, elderberry, rose hips, and licorice root are known for their immune-boosting properties, helping the body fend off infections and strengthen the immune system.
4. **Antioxidant Protection:** Herbal teas rich in antioxidants, such as green tea, rooibos, hibiscus, and turmeric, help combat oxidative stress, reduce inflammation, and support overall health.
5. **Sleep Support:** Herbs like valerian root, passionflower, and chamomile are popular choices for promoting restful sleep, easing insomnia, and improving sleep quality.
6. **Detoxification:** Certain herbs like dandelion root, nettle, burdock, and milk thistle support liver function, aid in detoxification, and assist the body in eliminating toxins.
7. **Respiratory Health:** Herbs such as thyme, eucalyptus, licorice, and marshmallow root can soothe respiratory discomfort, ease coughs, and support respiratory health.

**Popular Herbs for Herbal Teas and Infusions**

1. **Chamomile (Matricaria chamomilla):** Chamomile is renowned for its calming properties, making it a popular choice for promoting relaxation, reducing anxiety, and aiding sleep.
2. **Peppermint (Mentha piperita):** Peppermint is refreshing and aids digestion, relieves nausea, soothes headaches, and promotes overall well-being.
3. **Lavender (Lavandula angustifolia):** Lavender has a delightful floral aroma and calming effects, ideal for relaxation, stress relief, and improving sleep quality.
4. **Ginger (Zingiber officinale):** Ginger is warming, aids digestion, relieves nausea, reduces inflammation, and boosts immunity.
5. **Lemon Balm (Melissa officinalis):** Lemon balm has a refreshing citrusy flavor and is excellent for calming nerves, reducing anxiety, and improving mood.
6. **Echinacea (Echinacea purpurea):** Echinacea is well-known for its immune-boosting properties, helping the body fight off infections and colds.
7. **Rooibos (Aspalathus linearis):** Rooibos is caffeine-free and rich in antioxidants, making it a soothing and health-promoting beverage.
8. **Nettle (Urtica dioica):** Nettle is nutrient-rich and supports overall health, including immune function, skin health, and detoxification.
9. **Hibiscus (Hibiscus sabdariffa):** Hibiscus has a tart flavor and is loaded with antioxidants, supporting heart health, blood pressure regulation, and hydration.
10. **Turmeric (Curcuma longa):** Turmeric is anti-inflammatory,

antioxidant-rich, and supports joint health, digestion, and overall well-being.

**Brewing Herbal Teas and Infusions**

1. **Boil Water:** Bring fresh, filtered water to a boil. Use a kettle or pot for boiling water.
2. **Preparation:** Measure the desired amount of dried herbs, flowers, or spices based on your preference and the strength of flavor you desire.
3. **Steeping Time:** Different herbs require varying steeping times for optimal flavor and benefits. Generally, steep herbal teas for 5-10 minutes, but refer to specific guidelines for each herb.
4. **Infusion Techniques:** For herbal infusions, consider using a tea infuser, tea ball, or steeping directly in a pot and straining afterward. Infusions may require longer steeping times to extract flavors fully.
5. **Temperature:** Use the appropriate water temperature based on the herb or blend you're using. Some delicate herbs like chamomile and hibiscus may benefit from slightly cooler water (around 180°F or 82°C) to preserve their delicate flavors.
6. **Covering and Straining:** Cover the steeping vessel while the herbs infuse to retain aromas and flavors. After steeping, strain the herbal tea or infusion to remove solids and enjoy the liquid.

**Tips for Enjoying Herbal Teas and Infusions**

1. **Experiment with Blends:** Mix and match different

herbs, flowers, fruits, and spices to create unique herbal tea blends tailored to your taste preferences and health goals.

2. **Adjust Steeping Time:** Longer steeping times result in stronger flavors and more potent herbal infusions, while shorter steeping times may yield milder flavors.

3. **Sweetening:** If desired, sweeten herbal teas with natural sweeteners like honey, stevia, or agave syrup for added flavor.

4. **Iced Herbal Teas:** Enjoy herbal teas cold by refrigerating or adding ice cubes for a refreshing summer beverage.

5. **Herbal Tea Latte:** Create creamy herbal tea lattes by adding steamed milk or plant-based milk to brewed herbal teas for a comforting treat.

6. **Herbal Ice Cubes:** Freeze brewed herbal teas into ice cubes for adding flavor to water, iced teas, or cocktails.

## Safety Considerations and Precautions

- **Quality of Herbs:** Use high-quality, organic herbs free from pesticides or contaminants for optimal flavor and health benefits.
- **Allergies and Sensitivities:** Be aware of individual allergies or sensitivities to certain herbs. Start with small amounts and monitor for any adverse reactions.
- **Pregnancy and Medical Conditions:** Consult with a healthcare professional before using herbal teas, especially during pregnancy, breastfeeding, or if you have underlying health conditions or are taking medications.

## Conclusion

Herbal teas and infusions offer a delightful and health-promoting way to enjoy the benefits of herbs, flowers, fruits, and spices. From promoting relaxation and digestive support to boosting immunity and enhancing overall well-being, herbal beverages provide a wide range of flavors and health benefits. By exploring different herbs, experimenting with blends, and incorporating herbal teas and infusions into your daily routine, you can discover a world of aromatic, soothing, and flavorful beverages that nourish both body and soul. Remember to brew mindfully, prioritize quality ingredients, and savor the natural goodness of herbal teas and infusions for a healthier and more enjoyable lifestyle.

# Fifteen

# Integrating Herbal Remedies into Your Lifestyle

Integrating herbal remedies into your lifestyle offers a holistic approach to health and well-being, combining the wisdom of traditional herbal medicine with modern wellness practices. Whether you're looking to support specific health goals, promote overall wellness, or enhance self-care rituals, herbal remedies provide natural and effective solutions. In this chapter, we'll explore practical ways to incorporate herbal remedies into your daily life, from creating herbal first aid kits to cultivating herbal gardens and embracing herbal rituals for mind, body, and spirit.

## Creating Herbal First Aid Kits

One of the first steps in integrating herbal remedies into your lifestyle is to create a herbal first aid kit. A herbal first aid kit contains essential herbs, tinctures, oils, and salves that can address common health concerns and minor ailments. Here's how to get started:

1. **Identify Essential Herbs:** Select herbs that have versatile healing properties and can address a range of issues. Examples include calendula (for skin irritations), echinacea (for immune support), arnica (for bruises and sprains), and ginger (for digestive discomfort).
2. **Choose Herbal Preparations:** Stock your kit with various herbal preparations such as tinctures, infused oils, salves, teas, and dried herbs. These preparations offer different ways to administer herbs depending on the situation.
3. **Include Basic Supplies:** Don't forget to include basic supplies like bandages, gauze, cotton pads, tweezers, and scissors in your herbal first aid kit for comprehensive care.
4. **Educate Yourself:** Familiarize yourself with the uses, dosage, and administration of each herb and preparation in your kit. Keep a reference guide or book on herbal remedies handy.
5. **Organize and Maintain:** Keep your herbal first aid kit organized and easily accessible. Check expiration dates regularly and replenish supplies as needed.

**Cultivating Herbal Gardens**

Growing your own herbs is a rewarding way to integrate herbal remedies into your lifestyle while connecting with nature. Here are steps to cultivate your herbal garden:

1. **Choose Herbs:** Select herbs that thrive in your climate and are suitable for your needs. Popular culinary and medicinal herbs for gardens include basil, mint,

chamomile, lavender, thyme, and rosemary.

2. **Prepare the Soil:** Ensure your garden soil is well-draining, fertile, and free from contaminants. Amend the soil with compost or organic matter for optimal growth.

3. **Planting:** Plant herbs either directly in the ground or in containers based on space and preference. Provide adequate sunlight, water, and nutrients according to each herb's requirements.

4. **Harvesting:** Harvest herbs at the right time, typically in the morning after dew has dried but before the sun is too hot. Use sharp scissors or pruning shears to avoid damaging the plants.

5. **Drying and Preserving:** Dry harvested herbs for future use by hanging them upside down in a well-ventilated area or using a dehydrator. Store dried herbs in airtight containers away from heat and light.

**Incorporating Herbal Rituals**

Herbal rituals add depth and mindfulness to your daily routine, nurturing your mind, body, and spirit. Here are some herbal rituals to consider:

1. **Morning Herbal Infusions:** Start your day with a nourishing herbal infusion such as nettle, oatstraw, or tulsi (holy basil). These herbal teas provide nutrients, energy, and mental clarity.

2. **Herbal Baths:** Create relaxing herbal baths using dried herbs like lavender, chamomile, and rose petals. Add herbs to a muslin bag or directly to the bathwater for a soothing experience.

3. **Herbal Skincare:** Use herbal-infused oils or creams for skincare rituals. Calendula, chamomile, and rosehip oil are beneficial for soothing and nourishing the skin.
4. **Herbal Meditation:** Incorporate herbs like frankincense, sage, or cedar into your meditation practice. Burn herbal incense or use herbal sachets for aromatherapy during meditation sessions.
5. **Herbal Cooking:** Experiment with culinary herbs in your cooking to enhance flavor and nutrition. Fresh herbs like basil, cilantro, and parsley add vibrancy to dishes.

**Creating Herbal Remedies at Home**

Explore DIY herbal remedies to customize formulations based on your needs and preferences. Here are simple recipes to get you started:

1. **Herbal Tea Blend:** Mix dried chamomile, lavender, and lemon balm for a calming bedtime tea. Steep a teaspoon of the blend in hot water for 5-10 minutes and enjoy.
2. **Herbal Salve:** Infuse dried calendula petals in olive oil for several weeks, then strain and mix with melted beeswax to create a soothing herbal salve for minor skin irritations.
3. **Herbal Tincture:** Fill a glass jar with chopped ginger root and cover with vodka or brandy. Let it steep for 4-6 weeks, strain, and store in a dropper bottle for digestive support.
4. **Herbal Inhalation:** Boil water, add a few drops of essential oils like eucalyptus or peppermint, and inhale the steam with a towel over your head to clear sinuses and support respiratory health.

**Mindful Consumption and Dosage**

When integrating herbal remedies into your lifestyle, practice mindful consumption and dosage:

1. **Start Slow:** Begin with small doses of herbal remedies to gauge your body's response. Gradually increase dosage if needed while monitoring for any adverse reactions.
2. **Quality Matters:** Use high-quality herbs, preferably organic and sustainably sourced, for optimal potency and effectiveness.
3. **Consultation:** Consult with a qualified herbalist or healthcare professional, especially if you have specific health concerns, are pregnant or breastfeeding, or are taking medications.
4. **Listen to Your Body:** Pay attention to how your body responds to herbal remedies. Adjust dosage or formulations as needed based on your individual experience.

**Incorporating Herbal Wisdom**

Incorporating herbal wisdom into your lifestyle goes beyond using herbs for specific ailments. It involves cultivating a deeper connection with nature, embracing holistic wellness practices, and honoring traditional knowledge passed down through generations. Here are ways to integrate herbal wisdom into your life:

1. **Seasonal Alignment:** Align your herbal practices with the seasons. Choose herbs and rituals that support seasonal wellness, such as immune-boosting herbs in winter and cooling herbs in summer.
2. **Herbal Education:** Continuously expand your knowledge of herbalism through books, courses, workshops, and

learning from experienced herbalists. Deepen your understanding of plant properties, energetics, and therapeutic uses.

3. **Community Engagement:** Connect with herbal communities, local herb shops, farmers' markets, and herbalists in your area. Share experiences, exchange knowledge, and support sustainable herbal practices.

4. **Respectful Harvesting:** If harvesting herbs from the wild or your garden, practice sustainable harvesting techniques to ensure the preservation of plant populations and ecosystems.

5. **Gratitude and Ceremony:** Approach herbal practices with gratitude and reverence for the plants' healing gifts. Incorporate ceremonies or rituals to honor herbal allies and cultivate mindfulness.

## Conclusion

Integrating herbal remedies into your lifestyle is a journey of self-discovery, wellness, and connection with nature. Whether you're creating herbal first aid kits, cultivating herbal gardens, embracing herbal rituals, or crafting homemade remedies, each step brings you closer to holistic well-being and herbal wisdom. By incorporating herbal practices mindfully, respecting nature's gifts, and honoring traditional knowledge, you can enhance your quality of life, promote self-care, and embark on a meaningful herbal journey that nourishes body, mind, and spirit.

# Sixteen

# Conclusion

As we conclude our journey through the world of herbal health remedies, I invite you to reflect on the wisdom and insights you've gained, and the potential for transformation and healing that lies within your reach. Herbal medicine offers a holistic approach to wellness, drawing upon the healing power of nature to support our physical, emotional, and spiritual well-being.

In this book, we've explored a diverse array of herbs, their therapeutic properties, and practical applications for addressing common ailments and promoting overall health. From creating herbal first aid kits to cultivating herbal gardens, from crafting homemade remedies to embracing herbal rituals, each chapter has been a step towards greater understanding and empowerment.

As you incorporate herbal remedies into your lifestyle, remember that you are part of a timeless tradition that honors the interconnected-ness of all living beings. Whether you're sipping a soothing herbal tea, applying a healing herbal salve, or simply communing with nature in your garden, cherish each moment as an opportunity to nurture your body, mind, and spirit.

I encourage you to continue your exploration of herbal medicine, to deepen your knowledge, and to share your experiences with others. Together, we can cultivate a world where natural healing is embraced, and the wisdom of the plants is honored.

Thank you for embarking on this herbal journey with me. May your path be filled with health, vitality, and the abundant blessings of the natural world.

Wishing you wellness and joy,

Eric K. Williams

# Epilogue

As we reach the end of this journey through the world of herbal health remedies, I invite you to pause and reflect on the wisdom you've gained, the insights you've discovered, and the healing potential that lies within your grasp.

Herbal medicine is more than a collection of remedies; it's a way of life—a path to reconnecting with nature, honoring our bodies' innate wisdom, and embracing the holistic principles of well-being. Through the pages of this book, we've explored the healing properties of herbs, learned how to create herbal remedies, and discovered practical ways to integrate herbal wisdom into our daily lives.

As you continue your herbal journey, remember that the power of healing resides not just in the plants themselves, but in the intention and mindfulness with which we approach them. Whether you're brewing a soothing herbal tea, crafting a healing salve, or tending to your herbal garden, infuse each moment with gratitude, reverence, and presence.

May this book serve as a guide, a companion, and a source of inspiration on your path to wellness. May it empower you to take charge of your health, nurture your body and spirit, and cultivate a deeper connection to the natural world.

As we close this chapter, I extend my heartfelt gratitude to you, the reader, for embarking on this herbal journey with an open heart and a curious mind. May your herbal adventures continue to unfold, bringing health, vitality, and joy into your life.

With blessings and best wishes,
Eric K. Williams

# Afterword

As we come to the end of this exploration into herbal health remedies, I hope you have found inspiration, knowledge, and practical tools to enhance your well-being naturally. Herbal medicine is a vast and fascinating field, offering endless opportunities for learning, healing, and self-discovery.

In this book, we've delved into the therapeutic properties of various herbs, learned how to create herbal remedies, and explored ways to integrate herbal wisdom into our lifestyles. Whether you're seeking relief from a specific health issue, looking to support your overall wellness, or simply curious about the world of herbalism, I trust that you've found valuable information and insights within these pages.

As you continue your herbal journey, remember that healing is a holistic endeavor that encompasses not just the physical body but also the mind, emotions, and spirit. Take time to nurture all aspects of your being, listen to your body's wisdom, and trust in the healing power of nature.

I encourage you to stay curious, keep learning, and explore the endless possibilities that herbal medicine has to offer. Whether you're growing herbs in your garden, blending herbal teas in your kitchen, or crafting herbal remedies for yourself and your loved ones, know that you are part of a timeless tradition of natural healing.

Thank you for joining me on this herbal adventure. May your path be filled with health, vitality, and the abundant blessings of nature.

Warm regards,

Eric K. Williams